Sjögren's Syndrome Diet Cookbook

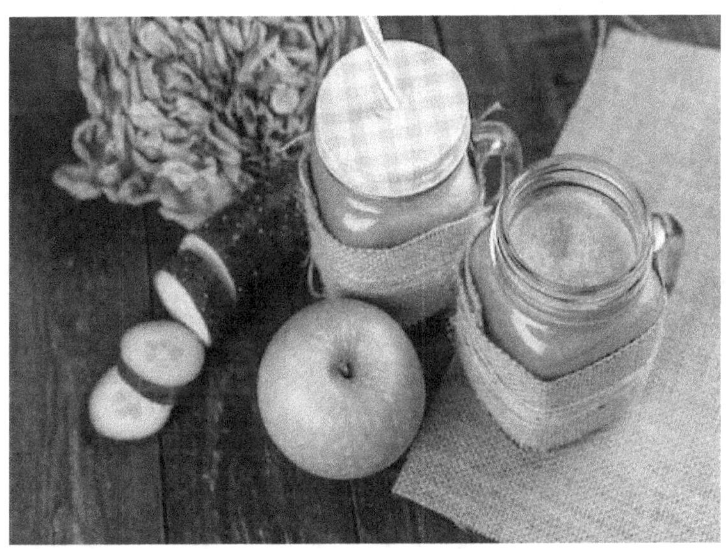

BENJAMIN THOMAS

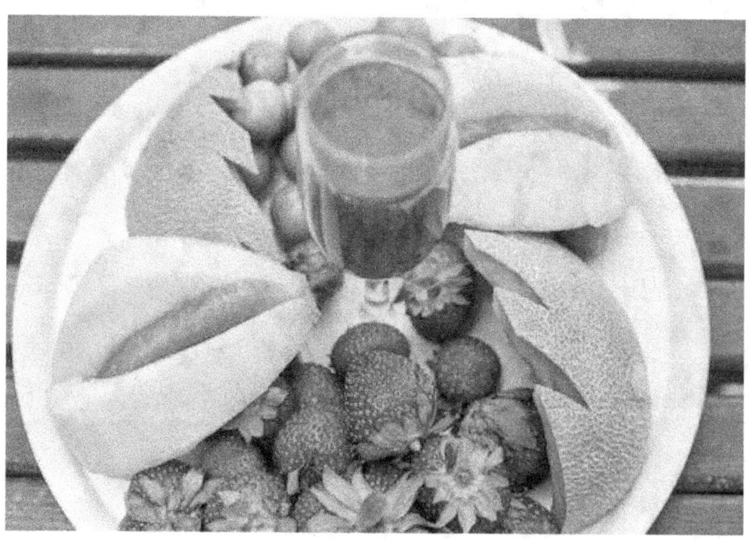

TABLE OF CONTENT

CHAPTER ONE

Introduction to Sjögren's Syndrome

Sjögren's Syndrome is a chronic autoimmune disorder characterized by the immune system attacking the body's moisture-producing glands, leading to a reduction in the production of saliva and tears. Named after Swedish ophthalmologist Henrik Sjögren, who first identified the condition in the early 20th century, this syndrome primarily affects the exocrine glands responsible for maintaining moisture in the eyes, mouth, and other mucous membranes.

One of the hallmark features of Sjögren's Syndrome is sicca syndrome, which manifests as dryness in the eyes and mouth. Beyond these primary symptoms, individuals with Sjögren's may also experience fatigue, joint pain, and inflammation affecting various organs, making it a systemic autoimmune condition. The prevalence of Sjögren's Syndrome is estimated to be around 0.1% to 0.6% of the global population, with a higher prevalence among women.

The exact cause of Sjögren's Syndrome remains elusive, but it is believed to involve a combination of genetic predisposition and environmental factors triggering an abnormal immune response. The condition can occur independently or coexist with other autoimmune disorders such as rheumatoid arthritis or lupus.

Living with Sjögren's Syndrome poses unique challenges, as individuals contend with not only the physical symptoms but also the potential impact on their quality of life. Dry eyes and mouth can lead to difficulties in swallowing, speaking, and increased susceptibility to dental issues.

Furthermore, the systemic nature of the syndrome may result in joint pain, fatigue, and a heightened risk of developing complications affecting vital organs.

While there is currently no cure for Sjögren's Syndrome, a multidisciplinary approach to management involves addressing symptoms, preventing complications, and improving overall well-being. This includes medications to alleviate dryness, manage inflammation, and, in some cases, immune-suppressive drugs. Lifestyle modifications, such as staying well-hydrated and managing stress, play a crucial role in enhancing the quality of life for individuals with Sjögren's. This cookbook is designed to provide practical dietary guidance and recipes tailored to support those managing the challenges of Sjögren's Syndrome, aiming to improve their nutritional well-being and overall health.

Common symptoms and challenges faced by individuals with Sjögren's.

Individuals with Sjögren's Syndrome face a myriad of symptoms and challenges that significantly impact their daily lives. The hallmark features of this autoimmune disorder include dryness, particularly in the eyes and mouth, known as sicca syndrome. Dry eyes can lead to irritation, a gritty sensation, and an increased susceptibility to eye infections. Concurrently, dry mouth, or xerostomia, poses challenges in speaking, swallowing, and can contribute to dental problems, such as cavities and gum disease.

Beyond the primary symptoms of dryness, individuals with Sjögren's often experience systemic manifestations affecting various organs and systems throughout the body. Joint pain and stiffness are common, resembling symptoms of rheumatoid arthritis.

This can hinder mobility and contribute to chronic discomfort, impacting overall quality of life. Fatigue is another prevalent symptom, often profound and unrelenting, leading to a sense of exhaustion that transcends normal tiredness.

The systemic nature of Sjögren's Syndrome can extend its effects to internal organs, potentially causing complications in the lungs, kidneys, and nervous system. Respiratory issues, such as chronic cough or shortness of breath, may arise, adding to the already challenging symptomatology.

In addition to the physical symptoms, individuals with Sjögren's face the psychological and emotional toll of living with a chronic autoimmune condition. Coping with persistent symptoms, managing medical appointments, and facing uncertainties about the progression of the disease can contribute to heightened stress and anxiety.

Moreover, Sjögren's Syndrome often coexists with other autoimmune disorders, further complicating the clinical picture and requiring a comprehensive and individualized approach to medical management.

The challenges of Sjögren's extend beyond the physiological realm, influencing various aspects of daily life, and necessitate a holistic care approach that addresses both the physical and emotional aspects of the condition.

This cookbook aims to provide practical dietary solutions to alleviate some of the challenges associated with Sjögren's, offering a path to improved nutritional well-being and enhanced overall health.

Impact of Diet on Sjögren's Syndrome Management

The impact of diet on managing Sjögren's Syndrome is profound, offering individuals an opportunity to mitigate symptoms and improve their overall quality of life. Given the chronic nature of this autoimmune disorder, adopting a carefully curated diet can play a pivotal role in addressing the challenges associated with dryness, inflammation, and systemic manifestations.

Hydration and Moisture Enhancement:

Maintaining adequate hydration is fundamental for individuals with Sjögren's Syndrome, particularly since the condition manifests as a reduction in the production of saliva and tears. Regular and sufficient water intake helps combat the effects of dry mouth and eyes, alleviating discomfort and promoting overall well-being. Including hydrating foods, such as water-rich fruits and vegetables, further supports moisture balance within the body.

Inflammation-Reducing Foods:

Inflammation is a key contributor to the symptoms experienced by individuals with Sjögren's. Adopting an anti-inflammatory diet rich in omega-3 fatty acids, found in fish, flaxseeds, and walnuts, can help reduce inflammation and alleviate joint pain associated with the syndrome. Antioxidant-rich foods, including colorful fruits and vegetables, combat oxidative stress and contribute to an anti-inflammatory environment within the body.

Avoidance of Trigger Foods:

Certain foods may exacerbate symptoms of Sjögren's Syndrome. For example, caffeine and alcohol can contribute to dehydration and worsen dryness. Spicy or acidic foods may irritate the mouth and eyes. By identifying and minimizing the consumption of trigger foods, individuals can better manage their symptoms and enhance their overall comfort.

Oral Health Support:

Dental issues, such as cavities and gum disease, are common challenges for individuals with Sjögren's due to reduced saliva production. A diet rich in calcium and vitamin D supports dental health by promoting strong teeth and bones. Incorporating foods like dairy products, leafy greens, and fortified plant-based milk can contribute to oral health maintenance.

Collaboration with Healthcare Professionals:

While dietary adjustments can positively impact symptom management, it is essential for individuals with Sjögren's to collaborate closely with healthcare professionals, including registered dietitians and rheumatologists. A personalized approach, considering the individual's overall health, nutritional needs, and potential medication interactions, ensures a comprehensive strategy for managing Sjögren's through diet.

This Cookbook's Contribution:

This cookbook is designed to complement medical management by offering practical and delicious recipes tailored to address the unique dietary needs of individuals with Sjögren's Syndrome. Emphasizing hydration, anti-inflammatory ingredients, and oral health support, these recipes aim to empower individuals to take an active role in their well-being through mindful and enjoyable eating practices.

Nutritional Considerations for Sjögren's Patients

Nutritional considerations for individuals with Sjögren's Syndrome are crucial for addressing the specific challenges associated with this autoimmune disorder. As Sjögren's primarily affects the moisture-producing glands, including those responsible for saliva and tears, a thoughtful approach to nutrition becomes essential to alleviate symptoms and enhance overall well-being.

Hydration is Key:

Given the hallmark dryness experienced by Sjögren's patients, maintaining optimal hydration is paramount. Adequate water intake helps counteract the effects of reduced saliva and tears, promoting moisture in the mouth and eyes. Incorporating hydrating foods, such as water-rich fruits like watermelon and cucumbers, can contribute to overall hydration levels.

Focus on Omega-3 Fatty Acids:

Inflammation is a common component of autoimmune disorders, including Sjögren's Syndrome. Omega-3 fatty acids, found in fatty fish like salmon, chia seeds, and flaxseeds, have anti-inflammatory properties that may help alleviate joint pain and inflammation associated with the syndrome. Including these foods in the diet can contribute to a more balanced inflammatory response.

Oral Health Supportive Nutrients:

Reduced saliva production in Sjögren's patients increases the risk of dental issues. Nutrients like calcium and vitamin D play a crucial role in maintaining strong teeth and bones. Dairy products, fortified plant-based milk, and leafy greens are excellent sources of these essential nutrients, supporting overall oral health.

Incorporating Anti-Inflammatory Foods:

A diet rich in anti-inflammatory foods can help manage systemic inflammation associated with Sjögren's Syndrome. Colorful fruits and vegetables, nuts, and seeds contain antioxidants that combat oxidative stress and contribute to a more balanced immune response.

Emphasis on Enjoyable Eating:

Maintaining a positive relationship with food is crucial for overall well-being. This cookbook is designed to make nutritional considerations for Sjögren's patients enjoyable and delicious. By incorporating flavorful and hydrating ingredients, the recipes aim to provide a practical and enjoyable way for individuals with Sjögren's to address their unique nutritional needs and enhance their overall health.

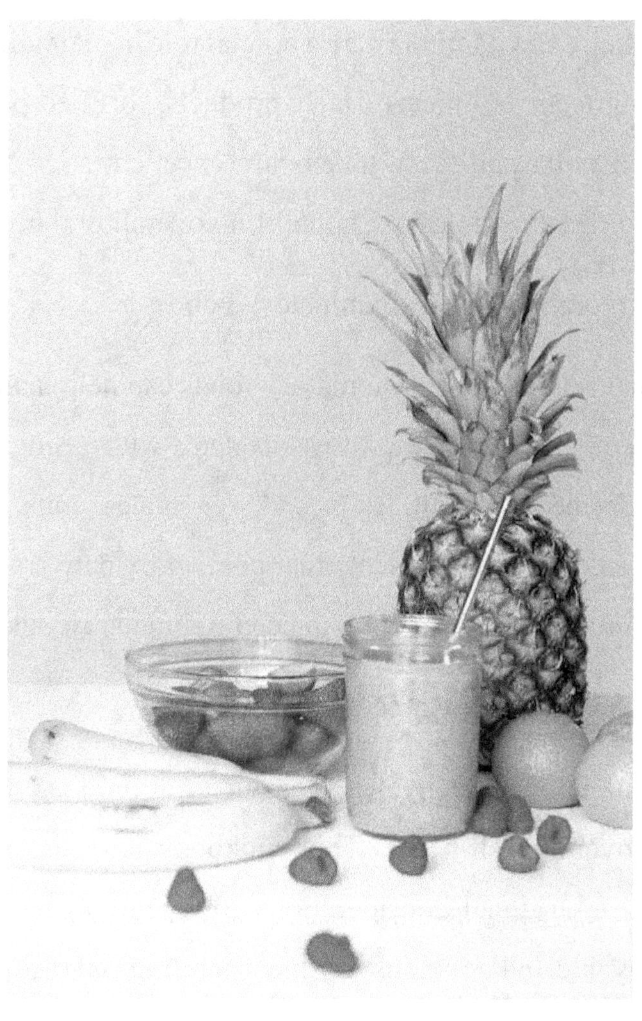

CHAPTER TWO

The Importance of Hydration for Sjögren's Patients

The importance of hydration holds immense significance for individuals grappling with Sjögren's Syndrome, a chronic autoimmune disorder characterized by the immune system's attack on moisture-producing glands.

As a condition primarily marked by dryness, especially in the eyes and mouth, maintaining optimal hydration becomes a cornerstone in managing the symptoms and enhancing the overall well-being of Sjögren's patients.

Combatting Dry Mouth:

Dry mouth, or xerostomia, is a prevalent and uncomfortable symptom for individuals with Sjögren's. Insufficient saliva production not only impacts the ability to speak and swallow but also heightens the risk of dental issues such as cavities and gum disease. Adequate hydration plays a pivotal role in mitigating dry mouth, as water helps compensate for the decreased saliva flow, providing relief and contributing to oral comfort.

Alleviating Dry Eyes:

Hydration is equally vital in addressing the dryness experienced in the eyes. Dry eyes can lead to irritation, a gritty sensation, and an increased susceptibility to infections. Drinking an ample amount of water supports tear production and helps maintain moisture on the ocular surface, reducing discomfort and supporting overall eye health.

Enhancing Moisture Throughout the Body:

Beyond addressing specific symptoms, hydration is crucial for sustaining moisture throughout the body. It helps maintain lubrication in joints, potentially alleviating joint pain and stiffness commonly associated with Sjögren's Syndrome. Adequate hydration also supports the skin, preventing excessive dryness and contributing to a more comfortable overall experience for individuals living with Sjögren's.

Hydrating Foods as Complementary Support:

In addition to plain water, the incorporation of hydrating foods can further support the moisture balance within the body. Foods with high water content, such as watermelon, cucumber, and celery, not only contribute to overall hydration but also provide essential nutrients that complement the dietary needs of individuals with Sjögren's.

Daily Hydration Goals:

Establishing and adhering to daily hydration goals is imperative for Sjögren's patients. It involves consistently consuming an adequate amount of water throughout the day, mindful of factors like climate and physical activity that may increase hydration needs.

The aim is to prevent dehydration, which can exacerbate the symptoms of dryness and contribute to an array of complications.

Holistic Approach to Well-being:

Emphasizing the importance of hydration in Sjögren's management underscores a holistic approach to well-being. Hydration is not merely a remedy for specific symptoms but an essential component of self-care that contributes to the overall comfort and quality of life for individuals navigating the challenges of Sjögren's Syndrome.

This cookbook integrates the significance of hydration into its recipes, offering enjoyable and hydrating culinary solutions to support individuals with Sjögren's in their daily lives.

Hydrating Foods and Beverages

Hydrating foods and beverages play a crucial role in supporting individuals with Sjögren's Syndrome, a chronic autoimmune disorder characterized by reduced moisture production in glands. Including foods with high water content and opting for hydrating beverages becomes a valuable dietary strategy to alleviate dryness and enhance overall well-being.

Hydrating Foods:

Cucumbers: Comprising over 95% water, cucumbers are not only refreshing but also contribute significantly to daily hydration needs.

Watermelon: With its juicy and succulent nature, watermelon is a hydrating fruit, offering a delicious way to increase fluid intake.

Celery: Known for its crisp texture, celery is rich in water and adds a hydrating crunch to salads and snacks.

Strawberries: Apart from being a vibrant and flavorful addition to meals, strawberries have high water content, contributing to hydration.

Melons: Varieties like cantaloupe and honeydew are excellent choices, packing both sweetness and hydration.

Hydrating Beverages:

Water: The simplest and most effective way to stay hydrated, water is essential for combating dryness in the mouth and eyes.

Coconut Water: A natural electrolyte-rich beverage, coconut water not only hydrates but also replenishes essential minerals.

Herbal Teas: Caffeine-free herbal teas, such as chamomile or peppermint, provide hydration along with potential calming effects.

Infused Water: Elevate plain water by infusing it with slices of fruits like citrus, berries, or cucumber for added flavor and hydration.

Broths and Soups: Clear broths and hydrating soups, especially those based on vegetables, contribute to fluid intake while offering nourishment.

Strategies for Hydration:

Consistent Sipping: Rather than consuming large amounts at once, frequent sips throughout the day help maintain hydration levels.

Mindful Snacking: Incorporating hydrating fruits and vegetables into snacks contributes to both nutrition and fluid intake.

Flavorful Hydration: Infusing water with natural flavors or opting for herbal teas makes hydrating more enjoyable.

By prioritizing hydrating foods and beverages, individuals with Sjögren's can proactively manage the challenges of dryness associated with the condition. This cookbook integrates these hydrating elements into its recipes, ensuring a delicious and practical approach to supporting hydration needs while embracing a diverse and enjoyable culinary experience.

Anti-Inflammatory Ingredients and Meals

Incorporating anti-inflammatory ingredients and meals into the diet is a valuable strategy for individuals managing Sjögren's Syndrome, an autoimmune disorder characterized by inflammation and reduced moisture production in glands. By choosing foods known for their anti-inflammatory properties, individuals can potentially alleviate joint pain, reduce inflammation, and enhance overall well-being.

Turmeric:

Curcumin, the active compound in turmeric, is renowned for its potent anti-inflammatory effects. Including turmeric in meals, such as curries or golden milk, can contribute to managing inflammation associated with Sjögren's.

Fatty Fish:

Rich in omega-3 fatty acids, fatty fish like salmon, mackerel, and trout possess anti-inflammatory properties. These fats help modulate the body's inflammatory response and may benefit individuals experiencing joint pain.

Leafy Greens:

Dark leafy greens, including kale, spinach, and Swiss chard, are abundant in vitamins, minerals, and antioxidants that combat oxidative stress and inflammation. Incorporating these greens into salads, smoothies, or cooked dishes can support overall health.

Berries:

Berries, such as blueberries, strawberries, and raspberries, are packed with antioxidants that help reduce inflammation. They offer a sweet and nutritious addition to meals, snacks, or desserts.

Ginger:

Ginger contains gingerol, a bioactive compound known for its anti-inflammatory and antioxidant properties. Adding fresh ginger to teas, stir-fries, or marinades can contribute to an anti-inflammatory diet.

Olive Oil:

Extra virgin olive oil is a rich source of monounsaturated fats and polyphenols with anti-inflammatory benefits. It serves as a healthy cooking oil and can be drizzled over salads or used in dressings.

Nuts and Seeds:

Almonds, walnuts, flaxseeds, and chia seeds are high in omega-3 fatty acids and antioxidants. Including a variety of nuts and seeds in the diet provides anti-inflammatory nutrients and adds texture to meals.

Colorful Vegetables:

Vibrant vegetables like bell peppers, tomatoes, and carrots contain phytonutrients with anti-inflammatory properties. Creating colorful, vegetable-rich dishes enhances both visual appeal and nutritional value.

Green Tea:

Green tea is loaded with catechins, powerful antioxidants that contribute to its anti-inflammatory effects. Enjoying green tea as a beverage or incorporating it into recipes provides a soothing and health-promoting option.

By emphasizing these anti-inflammatory ingredients in meals, individuals with Sjögren's can proactively address inflammation and potentially experience relief from associated symptoms. This cookbook integrates these ingredients into recipes, offering flavorful and health-supportive meals designed to enhance overall well-being for those managing Sjögren's Syndrome.

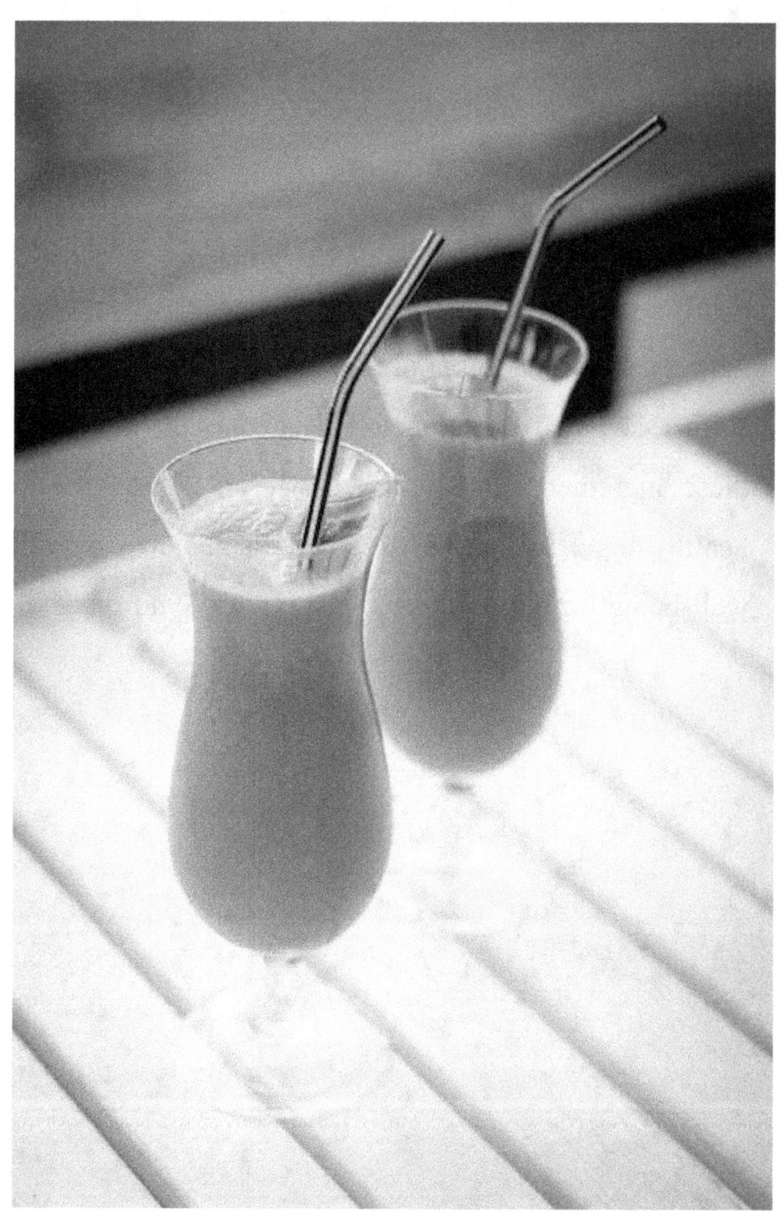

CHAPTER THREE

Sjögren's Syndrome Breakfast Diet Recipes

1. Hydrating Berry Smoothie Bowl

Ingredients:

- 1 cup mixed berries (blueberries, strawberries, raspberries)
- 1 ripe banana
- 1/2 cup Greek yogurt
- 1/4 cup almond milk
- 1 tablespoon chia seeds

Instructions:

- Blend mixed berries, banana, Greek yogurt, and almond milk until smooth.
- Pour the smoothie into a bowl.
- Top with chia seeds for added texture.
- Enjoy immediately.

Preparation Time: 5 minutes

2. Turmeric and Spinach Scrambled Eggs

Ingredients:

- 2 eggs
- 1 cup fresh spinach, chopped
- 1/2 teaspoon turmeric powder
- Salt and pepper to taste
- 1 teaspoon olive oil

Instructions:

- Whisk eggs in a bowl and add turmeric, salt, and pepper.
- Heat olive oil in a pan, add chopped spinach, and sauté until wilted.
- Pour the whisked eggs over the spinach and scramble until cooked.
- Serve hot.

Preparation Time: 10 minutes

3. Chia Seed Pudding Parfait

Ingredients:

- 3 tablespoons chia seeds
- 1 cup almond milk
- 1/2 teaspoon vanilla extract
- 1/4 cup granola
- Fresh berries for topping

Instructions:

- Mix chia seeds, almond milk, and vanilla extract in a jar. Refrigerate overnight.
- In the morning, layer chia pudding with granola and top with fresh berries.
- Serve chilled.

Preparation Time: 5 minutes (plus overnight chilling)

4. Omega-3 Rich Overnight Oats

Ingredients:

- 1/2 cup rolled oats
- 1/2 cup Greek yogurt

- 1/2 cup almond milk

- 1 tablespoon chia seeds

- 1/4 cup sliced almonds

- Fresh fruit for topping

Instructions:

- Combine oats, Greek yogurt, almond milk, and chia seeds in a jar. Mix well.

- Refrigerate overnight.

- In the morning, top with sliced almonds and fresh fruit.

Preparation Time: 5 minutes (plus overnight chilling)

5. Anti-Inflammatory Avocado Toast

Ingredients:

- 1 slice whole-grain bread

- 1/2 ripe avocado

- 1 teaspoon lemon juice

- Red pepper flakes for garnish

Instructions:

- Toast the bread slice.
- Mash the avocado and spread it over the toast.
- Drizzle with lemon juice and sprinkle red pepper flakes.
- Enjoy this flavorful and anti-inflammatory breakfast.

Preparation Time: 5 minutes

6. Green Tea Infused Quinoa Porridge

Ingredients:

- 1/2 cup quinoa, rinsed
- 1 cup green tea (brewed)
- 1/4 cup coconut milk
- 1 tablespoon honey
- Sliced kiwi for topping

Instructions:

- Cook quinoa in green tea according to package instructions.

- Stir in coconut milk and honey.

- Top with sliced kiwi before serving.

Preparation Time: 15 minutes

7. Hydrating Watermelon Salad

Ingredients:

- 2 cups diced watermelon

- 1/2 cucumber, diced

- 1 tablespoon fresh mint, chopped

- 1 tablespoon feta cheese (optional)

Instructions:

- Combine watermelon, cucumber, and mint in a bowl.

- Sprinkle with feta cheese if desired.

- Toss gently and enjoy this hydrating fruit salad.

Preparation Time: 10 minutes

8. Coconut Water and Berry Smoothie

Ingredients:

- 1 cup mixed berries (strawberries, blueberries, blackberries)
- 1/2 cup coconut water
- 1/2 cup Greek yogurt
- 1 tablespoon honey
- Ice cubes (optional)

Instructions:

- Blend mixed berries, coconut water, Greek yogurt, and honey until smooth.
- Add ice cubes if desired.
- Pour into a glass and savor this hydrating smoothie.
- Preparation Time: 5 minutes

9. Anti-Inflammatory Omelette

Ingredients:

- 2 eggs
- 1/4 cup diced bell peppers
- 1/4 cup spinach, chopped
- 1/4 teaspoon turmeric powder
- Salt and pepper to taste
- 1 teaspoon olive oil

Instructions:

- Whisk eggs and add turmeric, salt, and pepper.
- Heat olive oil in a pan, add bell peppers and spinach, and sauté until softened.
- Pour whisked eggs over the vegetables and cook until set.
- Fold and serve.

Preparation Time: 10 minutes

10. Honey-Sweetened Yogurt Parfait

Ingredients:

- 1 cup Greek yogurt
- 2 tablespoons honey
- 1/4 cup granola
- Fresh berries for topping

Instructions:

- In a glass, layer Greek yogurt with honey and granola.
- Top with fresh berries.
- Drizzle with additional honey if desired.

Preparation Time: 5 minutes

Sjögren's Syndrome Lunch Diet Recipes

1. Salmon and Avocado Wrap

Ingredients:

- 4 oz grilled salmon
- 1 whole-grain wrap
- 1/2 avocado, sliced
- Leafy greens
- 1 tablespoon Greek yogurt sauce

Instructions:

- Place grilled salmon, avocado slices, and leafy greens on the wrap.
- Drizzle with Greek yogurt sauce.
- Roll the wrap and enjoy.

Preparation Time: 15 minutes

2. Quinoa Salad with Chickpeas and Cucumber

Ingredients:

- 1 cup cooked quinoa
- 1/2 cup chickpeas, drained
- 1 cucumber, diced
- Cherry tomatoes, halved
- Fresh parsley, chopped
- Olive oil and lemon dressing

Instructions:

- Combine quinoa, chickpeas, cucumber, tomatoes, and parsley in a bowl.
- Drizzle with olive oil and lemon dressing.
- Toss gently and serve.

Preparation Time: 20 minutes

3. Mango and Shrimp Salad

Ingredients:

- 4 oz grilled shrimp
- Mixed salad greens
- 1 mango, diced
- Red onion, thinly sliced
- Avocado, sliced
- Lime vinaigrette dressing

Instructions:

- Arrange salad greens on a plate.
- Top with grilled shrimp, mango, red onion, and avocado.
- Drizzle with lime vinaigrette dressing.

Preparation Time: 15 minutes

4. Turmeric Chicken and Quinoa Bowl

Ingredients:

- 4 oz grilled turmeric-seasoned chicken
- 1 cup cooked quinoa
- Steamed broccoli florets
- Sliced carrots

- Tahini dressing

Instructions:

- Arrange quinoa, steamed broccoli, and sliced carrots in a bowl.
- Top with grilled turmeric chicken.
- Drizzle with tahini dressing.

Preparation Time: 25 minutes

5. Cucumber and Dill Greek Salad

Ingredients:

- 1 cucumber, diced
- Cherry tomatoes, halved
- Kalamata olives, sliced
- Feta cheese, crumbled
- Fresh dill, chopped
- Greek salad dressing

Instructions:

- Combine cucumber, tomatoes, olives, feta, and dill in a bowl.
- Drizzle with Greek salad dressing.
- Toss gently and serve.

Preparation Time: 15 minutes

6. Sesame Ginger Tofu Stir-Fry

Ingredients:

- 6 oz firm tofu, cubed
- Mixed stir-fry vegetables
- Brown rice, cooked
- Sesame ginger sauce

Instructions:

- Stir-fry tofu and mixed vegetables in a pan.
- Serve over cooked brown rice.
- Drizzle with sesame ginger sauce.

Preparation Time: 20 minutes

7. Caprese Salad with Balsamic Glaze

Ingredients:

- Fresh mozzarella, sliced
- Cherry tomatoes, halved
- Fresh basil leaves
- Balsamic glaze
- Olive oil
- Salt and pepper to taste

Instructions:

- Arrange mozzarella, cherry tomatoes, and basil on a plate.
- Drizzle with balsamic glaze and olive oil.
- Season with salt and pepper.

Preparation Time: 10 minutes

8. Sweet Potato and Chickpea Buddha Bowl

Ingredients:

- Roasted sweet potato cubes
- 1/2 cup cooked quinoa
- 1/2 cup chickpeas, roasted
- Sliced avocado
- Tahini-lemon dressing

Instructions:

- Assemble sweet potato, quinoa, chickpeas, and avocado in a bowl.
- Drizzle with tahini-lemon dressing.

Preparation Time: 30 minutes

9. Tomato Basil Zoodle Salad

Ingredients:

- Zucchini noodles (zoodles)
- Cherry tomatoes, halved

- Fresh basil leaves, torn

- Mozzarella balls

- Balsamic vinaigrette

Instructions:

- Toss zoodles, cherry tomatoes, basil, and mozzarella in a bowl.

- Drizzle with balsamic vinaigrette.

- Serve chilled.

Preparation Time: 15 minutes

10. Chicken and Vegetable Lettuce Wraps

Ingredients:

- Grilled chicken strips

- Butter lettuce leaves

- Julienne carrots and bell peppers

- Cilantro, chopped

- Hoisin-peanut sauce

Instructions:

- Place grilled chicken, carrots, bell peppers, and cilantro on lettuce leaves.
- Drizzle with hoisin-peanut sauce.
- Wrap and enjoy.

Preparation Time: 20 minutes

Sjögren's Syndrome Dinner Diet Recipes

1. Grilled Lemon Herb Chicken

Ingredients:

- 6 oz boneless, skinless chicken breast
- 1 lemon (juiced)
- Fresh herbs (rosemary, thyme)
- Olive oil
- Salt and pepper to taste

Instructions:

- Marinate chicken in lemon juice, fresh herbs, olive oil, salt, and pepper.
- Grill until cooked through.
- Serve with your favorite hydrating side vegetables.

Preparation Time: 30 minutes

2. Baked Salmon with Dill and Asparagus

Ingredients:

- 4 oz salmon fillet
- Fresh dill, chopped
- Lemon slices
- Asparagus spears
- Olive oil
- Salt and pepper to taste

Instructions:

- Preheat the oven. Place salmon on a baking sheet.
- Season with fresh dill, lemon slices, olive oil, salt, and pepper.
- Add asparagus around the salmon.
- Bake until salmon is cooked through.

Preparation Time: 25 minutes

3. Mushroom and Spinach Quinoa Risotto

Ingredients:

- 1 cup quinoa, cooked
- 1 cup mushrooms, sliced
- 2 cups fresh spinach
- Onion, diced
- Garlic, minced
- Vegetable broth
- Parmesan cheese (optional)

Instructions:

- Sauté mushrooms, onion, and garlic until tender.
- Add spinach and cook until wilted.
- Stir in cooked quinoa and vegetable broth.
- Cook until the liquid is absorbed.
- Top with Parmesan cheese if desired.

Preparation Time: 30 minutes

4. Turmeric Cauliflower and Chickpea Curry

Ingredients:

- 1 cup cauliflower florets
- 1/2 cup cooked chickpeas
- Coconut milk
- Turmeric powder
- Curry spices (cumin, coriander, garam masala)
- Basmati rice

Instructions:

- Cook cauliflower and chickpeas in coconut milk.
- Add turmeric, curry spices, and simmer until cauliflower is tender.
- Serve over basmati rice.

Preparation Time: 40 minutes

5. Sesame Ginger Glazed Tofu Stir-Fry

Ingredients:

- 6 oz firm tofu, cubed
- Mixed stir-fry vegetables
- Brown rice, cooked
- Sesame ginger sauce

Instructions:

- Stir-fry tofu and mixed vegetables until golden.
- Add sesame ginger sauce and toss.
- Serve over cooked brown rice.

Preparation Time: 25 minutes

6. Lemon Garlic Shrimp and Zucchini Noodles

Ingredients:

- 4 oz shrimp, peeled and deveined
- Zucchini noodles (zoodles)
- Lemon juice
- Garlic, minced
- Cherry tomatoes, halved
- Olive oil
- Fresh basil, chopped

Instructions:

- Sauté shrimp with garlic in olive oil until cooked.
- Add zucchini noodles and cherry tomatoes.
- Drizzle with lemon juice and top with fresh basil.

Preparation Time: 20 minutes

7. Vegetarian Stuffed Bell Peppers

Ingredients:

- Bell peppers, halved
- Quinoa, cooked
- Black beans, drained and rinsed
- Corn kernels
- Salsa
- Mexican cheese blend

Instructions:

- Mix cooked quinoa, black beans, corn, and salsa.
- Stuff bell peppers with the mixture.
- Top with cheese and bake until peppers are tender.

Preparation Time: 35 minutes

8. Pesto Zucchini Noodles with Cherry Tomatoes

Ingredients:

- Zucchini noodles (zoodles)
- Cherry tomatoes, halved
- Pesto sauce
- Pine nuts (optional)
- Parmesan cheese (optional)

Instructions:

- Sauté zucchini noodles and cherry tomatoes.
- Toss with pesto sauce.
- Garnish with pine nuts and Parmesan if desired.

Preparation Time: 15 minutes

9. Miso-Ginger Glazed Cod with Broccoli

Ingredients:

- 6 oz cod fillet

- Miso paste
- Fresh ginger, grated
- Soy sauce
- Broccoli florets
- Brown rice

Instructions:

- Mix miso paste, grated ginger, and soy sauce.
- Coat cod with the mixture and bake.
- Steam broccoli and serve with brown rice.

Preparation Time: 30 minutes

10. Butternut Squash and Sage Risotto

Ingredients:

- 1 cup Arborio rice
- Butternut squash, diced
- Fresh sage leaves
- Vegetable broth
- White wine (optional)

- Parmesan cheese (optional)

Instructions:

- Sauté Arborio rice, butternut squash, and sage.
- Add vegetable broth (and white wine if using) gradually.
- Stir until rice is creamy. Top with Parmesan if desired.

Preparation Time: 35 minutes

CONCLUSION

In closing, this cookbook offers a diverse array of delicious and health-supportive recipes meticulously crafted for those managing Sjögren's Syndrome. Emphasizing hydrating and anti-inflammatory ingredients, these meals aim to enhance well-being and enjoyment at the dinner table. Through flavorful combinations and thoughtful preparation, this collection serves as a culinary companion, providing not just nourishment but also a source of joy in every bite. Here's to vibrant health and the pleasure of mindful eat.

www.ingramcontent.com/pod-product-compliance
Lightning Source LLC
Chambersburg PA
CBHW070727260726

48660CB00007B/2755